THE LITTLE BOOK
OF CALM...
HAEMORRHOIDS

Published by Lulu.com

ISBN: 978-1-105-92467-5

Disclaimer: I am not a doctor or a health-care practitioner. Your decision to implement any of the recommendations I make in this book is your personal responsibility and if you have any doubts about their safety or contraindications then you should consult a licenced physician first. Always read all of the information leaflet accompanying any medication before administering it to yourself or others.

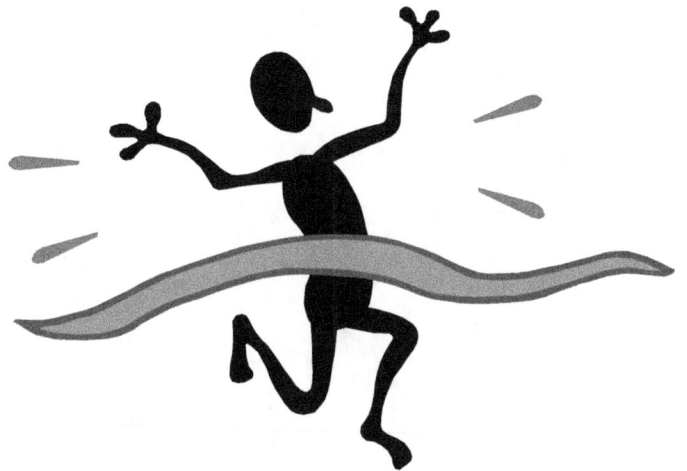

Call it what you like: anal varicose veins, haemorrhoids / hemorrhoids or piles, it's a horrible and sometimes excruciatingly painful condition and it makes the sufferer thoroughly miserable. In fact, I wouldn't be in the least bit surprised if marriages have been wrecked by haemorrhoids. Sometimes they're so painful they make even the most pleasant person grumpy and depressed. But as you're reading this book you probably know that already. What you want to know is how get rid of them. Well, not with homeopathy for a start. If you have succumbed, chuck it now. With a PhD and a background in scientific research my opinion of homeopathy is along the lines of 'exploitation of the desperate'. I prefer a dose of common sense, which I have relayed here in a simple step by step format and I sincerely hope it helps.

YOU ARE NOT ALONE

The first thing I must console you with is that you are *not* alone. It is estimated that fifty per cent of the population in the western world suffers from haemorrhoids at some point in their lives (though most would never dream of discussing it), and no, I am not going to subtly accuse either you or them of an unhealthy lifestyle. As well as constipation, some of the causes of haemorrhoids frequently listed are: exercise, pregnancy, genetics and plain old aging. I had always eaten plenty of fruit and vegetables and done masses of exercise and I still got haemorrhoids. I eventually got rid of them and then, two years later, I got food poisoning accompanied by a severe bout of diarrhoea and had to suffer and fight them again. The first time round it took me six months to win the battle, the second time, using the approach outlined in this book, it took me two to three weeks.

You are NOT alone and this is NOT your fault.

THE CATCH-22 OF GOING TO THE LOO

Haemorrhoids are basically caused by blood vessels in the anus either swelling or rupturing under pressure. The symptoms may include small protrusions from the anus, bleeding and anything from itching to intense pain. After the damage to the blood vessels has occurred it does heal but very, very slowly. The catch-22 is that just when it's starting to heal, you have to defecate again, which causes damage again, and so you fall into a vicious cycle which only leads to misery. Some people find that any form of movement after defecating just aggravates the pain, others find that sitting afterwards is painful. But the problem is that we are often forced to move around and / or sit (e.g. at a PC) in our daily lives: it can't be avoided. To cure haemorrhoids this vicious cycle must be broken.

A TWO PART
SOLUTION

The solution is twofold.

Firstly, to give haemorrhoids any chance of healing, re-damage to the blood vessels during defecation has got to be kept to an absolute minimum, and,

Secondly, defecation needs to be manipulated so that you have some control over *when* it happens and can lie down afterwards. The latter is tricky but possible.

But First,
A Note in Brief
On Pain Relief

If you're in pain right now, don't waste your time taking oral pain killers, they don't work. You need to directly apply pain relief ointment to the anus.

These ointments contain one of two active ingredients. Either the steroid cortisol (hydrocortisone) or the local anaesthetic lidocaine. I do not recommend hydrocortisone. It is well known to thin the skin which, in the case of haemorrhoids, just creates more bleeding (in my experience within a few days of regular application). It also does not provide immediate pain relief nearly as effectively as lidocaine-based ointments, such as Germoloids. Lidocaine-based ointments are *highly* effective at short-term pain relief, they are available off the shelf at the chemists and I thoroughly recommend them at the maximum daily dose.

If you need something right now, as a stopgap before you get to the chemists, an icepack might reduce the inflammation a little and may provide some brief relief. Then antiseptic cream rubbed on the anus does offer some lubrication to reduce the pain. You could also try a sitz (or saltwater) bath but, although it has sound theory behind it, it never worked for me.

Part I:

Minimising further damage to the Blood Vessels

Back then to the first aim—to minimise further damage to the blood vessels whilst defecating.

1. Finding the correct set of muscles

There are actually two different sets of muscles we can use to empty the bowels. The main set we use are the anus muscles, but they are the ones where the damaged blood vessels are and to heal your haemorrhoids you want to keep straining them to a minimum. It is also possible to evacuate your bowel by using a set of muscles higher up; the pelvic floor muscles. The best way to find these is to start by clenching your buttocks. You may have to experiment a bit to find them as you are probably not used to using them, I know I wasn't. Experiment with your position on the toilet: lean forwards, backwards and sideways; put your hands on the toilet rim; do anything to find out which position is the least painful. Some people find bringing their knees nearer to their chest helps and this is easily achieved by placing your feet on a low stool in front of the toilet.

There is, however, a major caveat—**you will *never* achieve evacuation of your bowels without the use of your anal muscles unless the faeces are incredibly soft** and loose. Let's face it, even if your thoughts right now are:

'But I've tried every position, every muscle, I don't understand what you're talking about and it still just plain HURTS.'

... then I completely understand. I didn't get it when I first read about it either. Even **if you don't understand what I've just written about different muscle sets, don't worry. All that matters is the looser the faeces are the less any muscles are going to be needed** and that can only be a good thing. So, the million dollar question is—How do you get the faeces loose enough to minimise further damage?

2. Eat fibre

Fibre absorbs water, so without plenty of fibre in your diet you won't achieve painless defecation. You may well have read this before but there is a lot more that you need to know, so read on.

Forget fruit and vegetables. They're good for you for plenty of other reasons but they're small fry compared to what you need right now. **You need foods with over 10 % fibre**. All-Bran is the best at around 25 % fibre, Bran Flakes are 14 % and porridge oats are 11%. A good wholemeal bread is around 8 % fibre. Once you get lower than about 8 % fibre content you're really fiddling with small change—it's not going to make the difference. For example, I have a bag of pears in my kitchen at the moment which are 2.2 % fibre. My New potatoes I notice are only 1.2 % fibre (yet the bag of oven chips in my freezer is 7.2 % fibre!) Fruit and vegetables may generally be higher in fibre than white rice and white bread, but they still contain *ten times* less fibre than All-Bran and Bran Flakes.

When you've got bad haemorrhoids you need two meals a day which are predominantly foods with over 10 % fibre. (I made them breakfast and supper).

3. All the fibre in the world is no use unless it's fully saturated _when it's in your bowel_

'But I eat tonnes of fibre and it still doesn't make any difference,' I hear you cry. I believe you. If it's a hot day and / or you are a lady menstruating you can drink pint after pint of fluid and, if your body needs it, it will absorb much of it from the food in your intestines, leaving barely any to reach all that fibre in your bowel.

I experimented extensively with fluid intake and there is only one way to saturate the fibre in your faeces with water before you defecate. That is to **drink 1–2 pints of hot water (e.g. as several large cups of tea) first thing in the morning when your stomach and upper intestine are completely empty** because you haven't eaten for around nine hours. This works like a dream. The liquid flows straight through you because there is no food present in the intestine to trap it. Your body doesn't have time to absorb it. Ninety per cent of the time this works within 15–20 minutes. If it doesn't then there probably just wasn't much in your bowels anyway, but the point is that what was there is now saturated with fluid. If you've eaten enough fibre this WILL work. (Have you ever wondered why Asian culture involves so much tea drinking despite the hot climate?)

4. It's softer, but it's not soft enough

If it still hurts, or if you are on holiday and haven't got access to high fibre foods, then **I strongly recommend a laxative**. Senna, which is a highly effective natural laxative, can be bought off the shelf at your local pharmacy (e.g. as Senokot) or the large supermarkets often do their own cheaper brands. You'll have to experiment to get the right dose for you—you don't want to overdo it. If you defecate more than once, or possibly twice, each day it can just further irritate the haemorrhoids (and you run the risk of dehydration and electrolyte deficiency associated with diarrhoea); it's a fine balancing act. I found that one tablet every 2–3 days helped and I have always made sure that I have some on holiday with me in case of an emergency since; especially in hot climates.

Never exceed the maximum dose given on the drug information sheet accompanying the laxative.

PART II:
CONTROLLING
WHEN YOU GO

Part I of this book will help you to reduce the pain during defecation. But it's still possible that you will encounter one of two problems:

1) While the pain has reduced, it still hurts, and more specifically it still hurts afterwards. Your haemorrhoids are irritated after going to the toilet and you've still got the whole working day ahead of you which is only going to aggravate them more. While your condition is not getting any worse, it's not getting any better either. You're in a kind of stalemate situation. Or,

2) You've got your bowels so loose that you're understandably concerned that you're going to lose control of them in an embarrassing situation.

At this stage you can get really down and miserable. It feels like this is going on forever. You've done everything you can and a nagging voice in the back of your mind says 'The only way to solve this is to starve myself for a few days'—DON'T! You've loosened the faeces; you're half way there. All you have to do now is find a way to control what time of day you defecate. It's tricky but it can be done.

The way to think about it is as follows: Night-time is healing time. When you wake up in the morning haemorrhoids aren't too bad. If you could delay defecating until late in the afternoon, just for one or two weeks, you would effectively be extending the healing time and severely reducing the throbbing, painful, damage-causing time to only a few hours in the evening. What is more, during those few evening hours, if you get yourself organised, you could just lie down.

There are two ways to do this. The first one is the easiest but you may need to do both in combination:

1) The laxative Senokot takes ~ 8–12 hours to take effect (I found it nearer to eight hours). So just take one first thing in the morning and it should take effect by the late afternoon. Obviously if you're using a different laxative the timing may be different.

2) Once you have faith in the hot morning drink flushing through you, why not delay it? Have a few small sugary drinks (e.g. fruit juices) and possibly a small breakfast, to keep you going through the day, then at about 3 pm start drinking your first pint of hot water. It can take up to two or three of these but by 4.30–5 pm it should have worked. **Then Eat!!** This is crucial. Eat as many calories as you would on a normal light-food day, just condense the hours of food consumption to between ~ 5 pm and bedtime. Particularly, have some supper. **If you don't you will never get through the next day.**

Whichever method you choose, for the rest of the evening lie down and read a book or watch TV. Do the absolute minimum you need to do.

I know this is difficult, and it can take a few days to work out how to successfully manipulate it, but it is worth persevering. It's only necessary for a week or so and then you should be comfortable enough to go back to a hot morning drink. But the hot morning drink I would personally make a habit for life.

[Note: obviously if your work routine is atypical, e.g. you work nights, you'll need to adjust the timings I have outlined but the same concepts still apply.]

IN SHORT...

✓ Get a lidocaine-based pain relief ointment and use it at the maximum dose.

✓ Experiment with both your position on the toilet and the muscle sets you use to defecate.

✓ Eat two small meals of very high fibre food (> 10 %) each day, e.g. Bran Flakes.

✓ To saturate that fibre, drink several pints of a hot water based drink **when your stomach is completely empty.**

✓ If you're still struggling, consider using a laxative such as Senna.

✓ Use the timing of the laxatives and the hot drinks to manipulate the time of defecation so that you can lie down afterwards.

A FEW OTHER THINGS THAT MIGHT HELP

1. After defecating wipe yourself with something soft (I used a damp piece of cotton wool) or shower yourself with a cool shower. (I always wondered what the deal was about bidets! Now I get it.)

2. Never hang on to go to the toilet. Go as soon as you feel a strong urge. If you leave it, the faeces just gathers into a large diameter at the base of your rectum which is harder to evacuate.

3. Don't keep straining on the toilet to get that last little bit of faeces out. In some cases suffers are actually detecting the haemorrhoids and mistaking them for faeces when there is nothing there. If there is a little left just leave it for next time.

4. Never wear underwear in bed or anything else that can rub haemorrhoids during the night. Healing during the night is your only chance of recovering, don't jeopardise it.

5. Ladies should remove tampons before defecating. They restrict full expansion of the anus when passing the faeces.

I sincerely hope this advice works for you.

If it doesn't work...

Go and see your doctor, don't live in pain. It's possible you have a different condition or that surgery is the best option for you. While recovery from surgery is reputed to be painful it's surely worth it if there is an end in sight?

If it does work...

Don't forget it! Tuck this book away somewhere safe just in case it happens again. Remember my food poisoning experience! Rubbing underwear can be another unforeseen culprit. Haemorrhoids can creep up on you so keep drinking your hot morning drink before breakfast and if you travel away from home always have a few laxatives tucked in your back pocket.

Good Luck.